Q&A on PKD

Scientific Advisory Board
of the
Polycystic Kidney Research
Foundation

Patricia A. Gabow, MD
Jared J. Grantham, MD

Editors

Polycystic Kidney Research Foundation

PKR Foundation
4901 Main Street, Suite 200
Kansas City, MO 64112
800-PKD-CURE
www.pkdcure.org

Printed in the United States of America by
The PKR Foundation

ISBN 0-9614567-2-8

Copy editors: Wendy Rueb, Deborah Hirsch

Q&A
on
PKD

---

an introduction

In four short years since we published the last *Q&A* book, laboratory and clinical research have produced significant breakthroughs in the diagnosis, treatment and understanding of polycystic kidney disease. We now stand on the threshold of developing a treatment and a cure for the predominant form of PKD.

With the recent identification of the PKD-1 gene, the localization of the ARPKD gene, the infantile type of PKD (to chromosome 6), and the promising use of drug agents to slow the progression of PKD in laboratory animals, we have every reason to believe that a treatment and cure are possible, hopefully during this generation.

While these breakthroughs are encouraging, what of those people who now have PKD? What does their future hold ... both short and long term? How do they better manage their day-to-day lives as PKD patients?

In an effort to summarize what we know about PKD and its effects on individuals and families, we are pleased to provide this new and revised version of *Q&A on PKD*. We trust it will be a particularly useful resource to anyone interested in knowing more about this prevalent, yet little known, disease. We also hope that, due to newer and greater advances in medical science, one day we can work ourselves out of a job and declare **"victory"** over PKD! That is our goal and the focus of everything we do!

Dan Larson
President, PKR Foundation
Third Edition

PKR Foundation
Scientific Advisory Board

The answers to the questions posed in this book should not be taken as specific advice to any individual. They represent consensus views of several physicians and may be subject to change as new knowledge is obtained.

Contents

v

PKD-1 Gene Identified

On June 17, 1994, the prestigious journal *Cell* reported that the long-awaited-for gene had been partially sequenced and verified as the cause of PKD-1.

Dr. Stephen Reeders, a past member of the PKRF Scientific Advisory Board, first localized the PKD-1 gene on chromosome 16 in 1985.

Four research teams in England, Wales, Portugal and the Netherlands worked in consortium after discovering a clue in chromosome 16 of a Portuguese family. In afflicted members of the family, the PKD-1 gene had been damaged by a break in the chromosome and the distal part of the chromosome had been exchanged with a chunk of chromosome 22. Additional mutations in this piece of DNA were sought in hundreds of other families with the autosomal dominant form of PKD, and three more were found that could impair the function of the gene.

1

ADPKD-1 accounts for approximately 85 percent of the cases of PKD that primarily affect adults. A second gene, ADPKD-2 that accounts for 10 percent to 15 percent of the cases, is known to exist, but the exact location on chromosome 4 has not been pinpointed.

Genetic researchers can now turn their attention to determining the abnormal protein encoded by the mutant gene, the next hurdle in understanding how this inherited disease causes cysts to form in the kidneys and other organs.

ARPKD Gene Located

The gene that causes devastating PKD in children is located on chromosome 6.

A group of European polycystic kidney researchers led by Dr. Klaus Zerres of Bonn, Germany, reported in the July issue of a leading scientific journal, *Nature Genetics,* that a gene for autosomal recessive polycystic kidney disease (ARPKD) had been mapped to chromosome 6. No other PKD genes are known to occur in this portion on the genome. This study required a high degree of cooperation among 14 scientists from 12 different institutions in Germany, France, Finland and Belgium.

ARPKD is one of the most common hereditary kidney disorders of childhood. Several hundred cases occur each year in the USA; the incidence is approximately one in every 10,000 births. The children are often born with severe kidney failure that causes death shortly after birth. Scarring also occurs in the livers of these patients. Approximately one-half to one-third survive the neonatal period and mature to adulthood.

Neither parent is aware that he or she carries the mutant gene that causes ARPKD. Consequently, the birth of an affected infant is usually the first sign of the problem. Routine prenatal screening by ultrasound testing picks up a few of the cases. Dialysis and transplantation in the first year of life have increased survival.

The new discovery should lead to more accurate forms of prenatal diagnosis. It is also a critical step toward

3

cloning the gene that causes ARPKD, determining the process by which cysts form in the kidneys and scar tissue is laid down in the liver. ARPKD is a disorder that may be responsive to "gene therapy," a process under development that replaces defective genetic material with normal DNA.

The PKR Foundation sponsors several research projects that are aimed at understanding how ARPKD progresses and at ways to improve treatment for children with this condition.

Types of ADPKD

Patricia A. Gabow, M.D.
University of Colorado Health Sciences Center

Until 1988 it was believed that all autosomal dominant polycystic kidney disease was caused by an abnormality in a single gene ... in fact, that is what we thought about dominantly inherited genetic disease in general. Well, we got a big surprise. Once Dr. Stephen Reeders and his group discovered the location of the ADPKD gene on chromosome 16 (ADPKD-1), it was possible to start testing ADPKD families for the gene. About the first 100 families that were tested all seemed to have the gene on chromosome 16. Then the surprise occurred.

A large family in Colorado and a family in Italy who definitely had ADPKD did not have the gene on chromosome 16 ... this meant that there must be at least two different gene defects that could produce the disease we called ADPKD. Since those two families were reported, a number of other families have been reported. However, it appears that among Caucasians of European origin, more than 85 percent of the ADPKD is due to the gene on chromosome 16. Other ethnic and racial groups have not been well studied to see if this distribution of gene type is the same in all populations. Until 1993 we did not know the location of the second gene. Now we know it is on chromosome 4 (ADPKD-2).

Once we found out that ADPKD could be caused by two different genes, it was logical to ask if the disease caused by the gene on chromosome 16 and the disease

5

caused by the gene on chromosome 4 looked different. In fact, it appears that they do have some differences. It seems that patients with ADPKD-2 are older when they first develop cysts, are older when they get hypertension, and go into end-stage renal disease (ESRD) at an older age. In one study the average age for reaching a serum creatinine of more than 1.5 mg/dl was 49 years in ADPKD-1 patients and older than 70 years in ADPKD-2 patients. There have been no studies looking at the frequency of the nonrenal abnormalities such as liver cysts or aneurysms in ADPKD-2, but these will be important questions. As if it weren't enough that ADPKD could be caused by two different genes, there is some preliminary evidence to suggest that there are ADPKD families whose gene is not on either chromosome 16 or 4. Will there be an ADPKD-3?

These are interesting genetic questions which, when answered, will help us understand how the disease actually occurs. It is also possible that classifying patients by the type of gene will help us better predict their clinical course.

Kidney Infection

William M. Bennett, M.D.
Oregon Health Sciences University

Infection involving the kidneys, particularly if cysts themselves are involved, can be a dangerous complication of ADPKD. This is rare, particularly if bladder infections, which are more common (particularly in women), are promptly diagnosed and treated.

The main symptoms of bladder infection are frequent urination with burning. Sometimes blood-tinged or foul smelling urine is noted, and oftentimes there is an urgency to void and a pressure feeling above the bladder—like you have to go right now! In women, keeping a full bladder all day at work, sexual intercourse without bladder emptying afterwards, and lack of fluid intake can all predispose to these infections. Fever is usually absent. Vaginal problems such as discharge and fungal infections can give similar symptoms and should be excluded. In men, the problem is somewhat less common, but prostate infection and abnormal emptying of the bladder are predisposing factors. Prompt institution of treatment with antibiotics of almost any type, plus increased fluid intake will eliminate the symptoms and signs of infection in a few days. Since bladder bacteria can ascend from the bladder to the kidneys, it is useful to identify the bacteria causing the infection by culture. However, treatment may be started before the culture results return. Any time the urinary tract is instrumented, like in passing a catheter, bacteria can be spread from the bladder up to the kidneys. You should notify your doctor that you have ADPKD prior to any procedure on the urinary tract. He or she may want to prescribe prophylactic antibiotics.

When the kidney itself is involved with infection there is usually fever, chills, flank or back pain, nausea and sometimes a feeling of severe illness. It is difficult to tell if the cysts are involved, so the doctor must remain vigilant for infections that are responding poorly to antibiotics. Usually hospitalization is required and, at least for a few days, antibiotics given by vein. Many antibiotics that treat kidney infections in other people do not work well in ADPKD patients because they do not penetrate the cysts. If this situation occurs, your doctor will have to decide whether to use a different drug that both penetrates cysts and is good against the particular bacteria that is causing your problem. Examples of these drugs are ciprofloxacin, trimethoprim-sulfamethoxazole and norfloxacin. These are scientific names, not brand names, which vary in different parts of the country.

To summarize:

1.   Seek medical attention promptly with urinary symptoms.

2.   Make sure all your doctors know you have ADPKD if they want to do any urinary tract procedures, and avoid instrumentation if possible.

3.   If you have a fever and it doesn't go away or if your symptoms persist, call the doctor again. You may need different treatment.

ARPKD and ADPKD in Children

Ellis D. Avner, M.D.
University of Washington

Both autosomal dominant polycystic kidney disease (ADPKD) and autosomal recessive polycystic kidney disease (ARPKD) can produce a variety of symptoms and clinical problems in affected children. The purpose of this review is to describe common clinical problems and their treatment in children with PKD.

Although ADPKD is generally thought of as a disease of adulthood, children who inherit one of the ADPKD genes (such as ADPKD-1 or ADPKD-2) from one of their parents may have a number of clinical problems since kidney cyst formation may begin even prior to birth.

9

Although uncommon, newborns with ADPKD can be born with massively enlarged kidneys, kidney failure, and underdeveloped lungs. Severely affected newborns may not be able to survive because their underdeveloped lungs cannot support their breathing. Others may have severely enlarged kidneys, but normal kidney function during early childhood.

Such infants may require special diets or feeding schedules to maximize their growth potential, and are commonly affected by hypertension.

Hypertension is far and away the most serious problem faced by children with ADPKD. Blood pressure control is of primary importance, not only to protect children from the immediate effects of hypertension (such as heart failure or stroke), but to also maximize long-term kidney function.

Blood in the urine is commonly seen when urine is examined under the microscope. However, unless grossly visible or accompanied by pain, this generally does not require any special study or treatment.

Abdominal or side pain may occur when a renal cyst enlarges, bleeds, is infected, or kidney drainage is blocked by a kidney stone. Ultrasound and other more specialized X-rays may be required to distinguish among these possibilities and guide specific therapy. In rare situations, surgical cyst reduction may improve complaints of chronic pain. Urinary tract infection can be a significant problem for children with ADPKD, particularly if complicated by infection of a kidney cyst. Regular monitoring of the urine and minimizing invasive urological procedures (such as urinary catheterization) can help to prevent infections in these children.

Preliminary reports appear to indicate that, like adults, children with ADPKD may have an increased incidence of cardiac valve abnormalities. Thus, any cardiac murmur in a child with ADPKD should be thoroughly evaluated by a pediatric cardiologist. The risk of cerebral aneurysms is fortunately quite rare in children with ADPKD. It is currently recommended that only children with strong family histories of cerebral aneurysms, otherwise unexplained headaches, or focal neurological symptoms undergo formal evaluation for this complication.

The appearance of cysts in other organs (such as the

liver or pancreas) in children with ADPKD is rare. Even when present, such cysts are generally small and cause no specific clinical problems. The majority of children with ADPKD have no symptoms whatsoever. In this group, regular monitoring of blood pressure and periodic kidney ultrasounds are the only measures needed for preventative health maintenance.

Children with ARPKD have symptoms quite similar to those noted above for children with ADPKD. In this condition, a child has received an affected gene from both of his/her clinically normal parents. Newborns may be severely affected and not survive the neonatal period. Enlarged kidneys and hypertension are quite common and need to be monitored and treated to prevent serious complications. An additional problem faced by children with ARPKD is portal hypertension. This is caused by scarring in particular areas of the liver, which block blood flow to that organ. This leads to abdominal swelling, enlargement of the spleen, and an increased risk of bleeding from enlarged abdominal blood vessels.

11

In children with ARPKD who develop such problems, a surgical procedure to re-route blood flow around the engorged liver may be necessary. An additional liver problem in children with ARPKD is infection of the liver drainage system (ascending cholangitis), which is characterized by fever and pain in the right upper abdomen. Although children with ARPKD may often have white blood cells present in their urine due to the structural changes in their kidneys, urinary tract infections do not pose a particular problem for them.

Both children with ADPKD and ARPKD can develop varying degrees of kidney failure. Kidney function in all such children needs to be monitored regularly. In many patients, phosphate binding medications (such as calcium carbonate), vitamin D, erythropoietin, and growth hormone, as well as aggressive nutritional support may be required to maximize growth and development. Ultimately, children with ADPKD or ARPKD may require renal replacement therapy with dialysis and/or transplantation. New improvements in dialysis and transplant technology mean that even infants can be successfully treated in special pediatric referral centers.

Although children with ADPKD and ARPKD may have a variety of clinical problems, the outlook for such children is quite promising if they are monitored and treated. It is strongly recommended that all children with ADPKD or ARPKD be referred to a pediatric nephrologist to minimize complications of their disease and maximize their ultimate rehabilitation.

Polycystic Kidney Disease in Adults

Diagnosis

Question: During the late 19th and early 20th centuries, what medical diagnoses of the cause of death or final illness would have been likely for persons who died with polycystic kidney disease? This is important to those of us who want to trace the family history of PKD.
College Station, TX

Answer: Before the modern era of sonograms, CAT and MRI scans, diseases such as ADPKD were often diagnosed as "uremic poisoning," Bright's Disease or Dropsy. Such diagnoses could be caused by a variety of kidney disorders, ADPKD among them. Terminal renal diseases are uncommon enough in the population at large that one of the above diagnoses would likely indicate ADPKD in a member of a family in which others had been identified with the disease. Other possible indicators include cerebral aneurysm and sub-arachnoid hemorrhage; enlarged kidneys might be mistaken for kidney cancer if they were not examined directly.

Question: There is a strong pattern of PKD in my family. At age 18 I was told (after kidney X-rays) that I did *not* have PKD. There is confusion in our family about who will and who will not have this disease in later life, even if an initial exam proved negative, as in my case. I am 28 years old. Arlington, VA

Answer: PKD has a variable age of onset, but in general most patients with the adult form of PKD will show X-ray signs at age 18, even if they have no symptoms. The standard dye test (IVP) that you probably had is the least sensitive of the tests now available.

In most centers, ultrasound (sonography) is sensitive enough to detect most cases of PKD, but not sensitive enough, in the view of most specialists, to completely exclude the diagnosis. The computed tomogram (CT scan) combined with dye infusion is the most sensitive test available. If at age 28 you have a negative sonogram and CT scan, current data indicates you do not have PKD and will not pass it on.

14

Question: In June 1986, I was diagnosed by CT scan as having PKD. Both of my parents had ultrasound tests to determine which one of them had PKD. Both of the ultrasound tests were normal. My question is: Are there ways to get PKD other than through your parents? Omaha, NE

Answer: To be absolutely certain that neither parent has polycystic kidney disease, a special CT scan with contrast enhancement would have to be performed on each of them. There are at least three reasons why a patient may show up with polycystic kidney disease and have neither parent show evidence of PKD.

First, the patient may represent a new mutation. What this means is the defective chromosome may have developed spontaneously rather than having been received from a parent. If the patient has a brother or sister with PKD or other relatives such as aunts, uncles or cousins with PKD, it is unlikely that the patient has PKD because of a new mutation.

Another reason, and this is a most sensitive issue, is the possibility that the patient is the product of different biological parents. Finally, the patient may have autosomal recessive polycystic kidney disease (ARPKD) rather than autosomal dominant PKD (ADPKD). To resolve this, careful history, physical and X-ray examination must be done in conjunction with a nephrologist.

Question: Is there a test available to determine if an unborn child has PKD? New York, NY

Answer: Researchers have used an alpha-globin marker to locate on chromosome 16 the gene that causes PKD. It would be possible to use the alpha-globin marker to look for the defective gene in cells from amniotic fluid, but the alpha-globin marker has an error rate that is not yet optimal for in-utero diagnosis. Researchers have found markers closer to the gene than alpha-globin.

Question: My doctor asked me to try and find out why some kidneys are so small in certain polycystic kidney patients and huge in others. Gibson City, IL

Answer: The observations are quite correct and the honest answer to the question is that no one knows. Not everyone with polycystic kidney disease has enlarged kidneys, although the majority do. The critical issue is the extent to which the cysts replace the normal kidney tissue. A few cysts in a normal-sized kidney will cause no difficulty. A multitude of cysts in a normal-sized kidney can do just as much harm as many large cysts in a greatly enlarged kidney.

Question: If PKD is such a common hereditary kidney disease, why is it that I have only talked to one person who actually has the disease and everyone else I have talked to has never heard of it? Medford, OR

Answer: Good question! One of the mysteries of PKD is why so few have ever heard of this condition. It is much more common than cystic fibrosis, sickle cell anemia and Down's syndrome, conditions that Americans are much more aware of than PKD. Your question affirms one of the important goals of the PKR Foundation, which is to increase the awareness of PKD among laypersons.

Question: I have PKD but my sister does not have it. She is interested in genetic counseling and her question is: Can PKD skip a generation? Fairhaven, MI

Answer: If your sister is over 25 years of age and does not have cysts in the kidneys and liver when examined by computed tomography scan (CT scan) with contrast enhancement, it is most unlikely that she has PKD. There are no documented instances to our knowledge that PKD has skipped a generation. In other words, if your sister does not have PKD at age 25, there is very little chance that her offspring will have the disease, provided of course that her husband does not have PKD.

Question: I understand that there is a blood test for all family members of a PKD patient to determine who else in the family has PKD and/or to determine which family member is a potential donor. Please provide more information about the test. Dayton, OH

Answer: A test is commercially available that depends on the linkage of PKD to a marker known to occur on chromosome 16. In order for the test to be informative, one must have one and preferably two or more living family members available who have the disease in order to determine which asymptomatic subjects in the family have the PKD gene. If you are interested in being tested, you can contact the genetics department of medical schools in your area, or you can write to the National Center for Education in Maternal and Child Health, 3520 Prospect St. N.W., Washington, D.C. 20057 and request a copy of its pamphlet entitled, "Comprehensive Clinical Genetic Services Centers: a national directory." This is a listing of genetic service centers throughout the United States which provide comprehensive diagnostic services, medical management, counseling and follow-up care.

Question: My husband has PKD and a 14-year-old daughter by his first marriage. I feel that with the problems my husband is currently having, she should be checked early in life. I would appreciate your suggestions. Barnsdall, OK

Answer: Most nephrologists no longer advise that parents check asymptomatic children for PKD until the child has reached the age of 18 and can legally make their own decision. If a child develops urinary tract symptoms at any age, appropriate diagnostic studies should be done to investigate the problem. There is no specific therapy to offer asymptomatic individuals with PKD. Therefore, the only reason to establish an early diagnosis is for genetic counseling and family planning. Too often, parents have made premature decisions for their children only to wish later that they had waited. There simply are no hard and fast rules in respect to your question. In any respect, presymptomatic testing in children should not be done without a great deal of thought, and when available, counseling with a knowledgeable genetic counselor and a nephrologist is indicated.

Question: My mother has polycystic kidneys as does my sister. I have a polycystic liver, and one polycystic kidney was removed because of infection. The remaining kidney is O.K. Do I have PKD, since only one kidney seems to be involved? Red Bank, NJ

Answer: In view of the strong family history and the evidence of cysts in the liver and one kidney, there seems to be little doubt that you have the hereditary form of PKD. There are a few reports of "one-sided" PKD in the medical literature, but these are extremely rare. A CT scan of the remaining kidney would resolve the issue.

Question: Do you believe that it is possible for me to be the only child of nine who has PKD? Chesterfield, NH

Answer: In each child of an affected parent, autosomal dominant polycystic kidney disease is a 50/50 proposition. It is like flipping pennies. Occasionally three, four, or five or more heads will turn up in a row. If one flips the pennies a sufficient number of times, the odds will always even out 50 percent heads, 50 percent tails. Many families seem to have a lopsided experience with polycystic kidney disease. In your case, it is a low statistical probability that you are the only one of nine children who has the disease, but not an impossibility. We have communicated with other families in which nearly all of the members seem to have polycystic kidney disease and only a few escaped without it. Large-scale studies of many PKD families have always confirmed the 50/50 ratio.

Question: I have PKD and am of Polish-Jewish background. Do you know if there are certain ethnic groups more prone to developing PKD? Kinnelon, NJ

Answer: PKD is found on all continents, in all races and in all ethnic groups. No information has become available to suggest that one social group may have a different prevalence of PKD than another. This is a question that should be resolved in the next few years as researchers do a better job of studying the epidemiologic patterns of all renal diseases.

Question: Though the gene of polycystic kidney disease is autosomal dominant, isn't there occasionally incomplete penetrance? West Lafayette, IN

Answer: In dominantly inherited diseases, 50 percent of the offspring of an affected parent may inherit the defective gene. If the disease is dominant, then it should be seen in all patients who have the defective gene. In a number of studies (done by perfoming radiographic studies on all patients at risk for PKD whether they had symptoms of the disease or not), ADPKD has been clearly shown to be an autosomal dominant condition. Incomplete penetrance is a term used to describe a genetic disorder that does not always show up in every sequential generation of a family. Incompletely penetrant genes cause the particular disease to "skip" generations. ADPKD appears to "skip" generations in some families but incomplete penetrance is not the reason why. If sensitive radiographic tests are not performed, some subjects who have the ADPKD gene and a mild form of the disease may never become aware that they have it. They can, however, pass the gene on to their offspring, and it may resurface there. Thus, because ADPKD has mild forms of presentation in some individu-

19

als, it has incorrectly been grouped by some doctors among incompletely penetrant genetic disorders.

Question: You indicate in PKR updates that a milder form of PKD exists. I would like to know if a nephrologist can order a test to determine which form of PKD an individual has? Morristown, NJ

Answer: Two genetic types of autosomal dominant PKD are now recognized. PKD-1 affects the vast majority of individuals who have polycystic kidneys. Another genetic form, now called PKD-2, appears to have a milder clinical course than PKD-1. There is a genetic test available for the PKD-1 type, but it requires the participation of at least two affected individuals in the family along with the individual who is at risk. These tests are performed at only a few centers scattered throughout the United States. With the recent mapping of the PKD-2 gene on chromosome 4, a similar type of testing for the PKD-2 type is now possible.

Hypertension

Question: My blood pressure is 145/100 and my doctor has recommended enalapril, which may help preserve kidney function as well as lower blood pressure as I understand it. Ithaca, NY

Answer: It is very important to bring blood pressure under good control as this will diminish scarring of the tiny blood vessels in the kidneys. Enalapril has been used for blood pressure control in polycystic patients with reasonable success. It is usually prescribed together with a salt restricted diet and weight control.

We do not know for sure if enalapril or other related drugs that block the angiotensin-converting enzyme have any other special actions for polycystic kidneys, but one hypothesis suggests that by lowering the blood pressure in the kidney filters (called glomeruli), we may prevent additional scarring of these important structures.

Confirmation of the hypotheses will not be known for several years, but, in the meantime, enalapril and other equally good blood pressure lowering drugs make good sense in the management of high blood presssure.

Question: I read the newsletter and mentioned to my doctor that patients with PKD were now taking cnalapril and captopril as treatment for hypertension. My doctor said that these drugs should not be used in patients who have renal failure, whether it is mild or severe. Would you please explain? Port St. Lucie, FL

Answer: These drugs can be used in patients who have mild renal insufficiency, but their use must be monitored carefully by the physician. Many patients with mild levels of renal insufficiency are being treated with these drugs. Occasionally when therapy is started there may be a slight decrease in kidney function reflected in an increase in serum creatinine level. Nephrologists are accustomed to dealing with these fluctuations in kidney function and should be able to alter dosage schedules to get an optimum effect on blood pressure with a minimal risk to kidney function. The potassium level should be monitored carefully in patients receiving these new drugs.

Question: I have ADPKD and was found to have hypertension in 1979. I have been treated with a combination of metoprolol and hydroclorothiazide, which has kept my blood pressure stable at 120/90. I have never realized side effects. My lab values are completely normal. I would like to know whether an ACE inhibitor (enalapril, captopril) would have any advantages in relation to my present pharmacologic treatment in this stage of my hypertension. Republic of Germany

Answer: Hypertension can accelerate the progression of renal insufficiency in patients with polycystic kidney disease. There is reason to think that ACE inhibitors may have a theoretical advantage in the treatment of hypertension in patients with ADPKD. A controlled clinical study has not been done, however, and we would not be inclined to recommend a change in treatment if the blood pressure is well controlled with the current regimen. On the other hand, in patients with hypertension who have not been previously treated, ACE inhibitors are probably good choices for the initiation of antihypertensive therapy.

Liver

Question: I have recently been found to have polycystic kidney disease with a polycystic liver. Is there anything I can do to help extend the life of my liver? Lincoln, NE

Answer: Polycystic liver occurs in approximately 40 percent to 60 percent of patients with polycystic kidney disease. Fortunately polycystic liver disease rarely causes the liver to fail, although in a few cases the liver can enlarge to a fairly great extent and cause problems because of its size.

We suggest that patients with polycystic kidneys and polycystic livers refrain from caffeinated beverages such as coffee, tea, and certain cold drinks. Recent experimental evidence in laboratory models of PKD indicate that the caffeine may conceivably cause kidney and liver cysts to expand at a faster rate than usual.

23

Question: I (female) have been told that I have cysts in my liver. I am 46, feel great except for the liver, which has grown quite a bit, and sometimes there is pain. There isn't much information about the liver in PKD. What can I expect? Ontario, CA

Answer: Liver cysts tend to develop later in life than renal cysts and are very rare before age twenty. Although men and women are just as likely to have liver cysts, many liver cysts and very enlarged livers are much more common in women with ADPKD than men. Women who have been pregnant are more likely to have liver cysts than women who have not been pregnant, and the occurrence of any pregnancy and the number of pregnancies influence the number and size of the liver cysts. If the liver becomes very large and causes severe pain or interferes with eating and daily activity, the liver cysts can be drained. If only one or two large cysts are causing the problem, they can be drained with a needle. If there are many cysts, surgery is necessary to drain or remove the cysts.

Question: I have large liver cysts that cause pressure on my upper waist and make me feel short of breath. I take a calcium blocker and nitroglycerin for my heart. Do either of these drugs make cysts grow faster? Geneva, NY

Answer: You raise an important general question for which we have almost no data. We suspect that caffeine and theophylline may increase the rate that cysts enlarge in the kidneys and the liver, but we have no information on the drugs that concern you the most.

24

Question: What is the usual treatment for extremely large (sometimes painful) liver cysts? Are medications helpful? PKRF Annual Conference

Answer: Most liver cysts do not cause symptoms and require no treatment. Rarely, one or a few liver cysts may become very large and cause a number of problems such as pain, sensation of fullness, heartburn, and shortness of breath. Medications that reduce the secretion of acid in the stomach and suppress the release of a hormone that stimulates the secretion of fluid into liver cysts may help some of these symptoms, but they are not likely to make the cysts smaller.

A large liver cyst can be drained through a thin tubing placed by a radiologist using ultrasound or computed tomography. If nothing else is done, the fluid usually reaccumulates within a few days, but injection into the cyst of one of a number of substances called sclerosing agents often results in long lasting reduction in size or even disapperance. Alcohol is the most commonly used sclerosing agent. Recently, laparoscopic surgery has been used to treat large liver cysts. In this procedure, which requires general anesthesia, the surgeon examines and works on the liver using a laparoscope (a narrow, flexible, fiberoptic tube) and surgical tools placed through small holes in the abdominal wall. Since no surgical incision of the abdomen is made, the recovery is very fast. Presently, the experience with laparoscopic surgery for the treatment of hepatic cysts is still very limited. Neither alcohol sclerosis nor laparoscopic surgery is helpful to treat patients with massive enlargement caused by many small- or medium-sized cysts. When these patients have symptoms severe enough to justify an invasive type of treatment, extensive surgical resection or, very rarely, liver transplantation may need to be considered.

Infection

Question: Is aspiration of a single large cyst indicated for relief of recurrent urinary infection? Atlanta, GA

Answer: There are multiple types of cysts that are not part of the genetic disease, polycystic kidney disease. Oftentimes, cysts can be causing obstruction in the urinary tract, which predisposes to infection, or, alternatively, infections may have nothing to do with the cysts at all since solitary cysts are common in the general population. A physician should evaluate each case so as to decide whether autosomal dominant polycystic kidney disease is present. In ADPKD, aspiration of single cysts is not routinely recommended unless severe pain or refractory infection is present. If another kind of cystic disease is present, the physician will need to determine what relationship that cyst has to recurrent urinary tract infections. If a single cyst is causing obstruction, it can be aspirated under ultrasound guidance and relief of pain symptoms may be obtained.

Question: Antibiotics help recurrent kidney infections for a few days, but the symptoms—nausea, fever, chills, pain, fatigue and weakness—recur when they are discontinued. My doctor is open to suggestions. Mesa, AZ

Answer: Recurrent kidney infections usually mean that one or more cysts have been infected. It is important for the physician to try to culture the bacteria from the blood-stream and the urine so that a specific treatment can be prescribed. Unfortunately, the bacteria "hide out" in the cysts and cannot be cultured in many cases, and antibiotics must be given blindly. We have known several patients who required continuous antibiotic treatment for several *years* in order to control the symptoms.

Research supported by the PKR Foundation has led to the discovery of two drugs that may be helpful in some patients with recurrent and resistant kidney cyst infections. One of them, chloramphenicol, is an old-time medicine that works well, but has a reputation for causing serious anemia on rare occasions. Nonetheless, it can be used for treating difficult cyst infections if patients are willing to take the small risk. Gyrase inhibitors (norfoxacin and ciprofloxacin) are very good for treating infected cysts. Considerable experience has been gained with these drugs, and so far only a few problems have surfaced.

Question: I am a 26-year-old female who has had three urinary tract infections in the last two months. My back has really been bothering me. Ladson, SC

Answer: Recurrent urinary tract infection is a very common problem for women, and especially difficult for PKD patients. Most often the bacteria (germs) that cause these infections enter the urinary tract through the urethra, the opening to the bladder just below the pubic bone. Many women can relate the infections to recent sexual intercourse. For patients with PKD, it is very important that a urine culture be obtained each time you have symptoms of infection (burning on urination, a feeling of urgency to pass urine, fever, chills, and back pain that develops with these other symptoms). The culture should be done by your doctor *before* you receive antibiotic treatment. Very often the infecting bacteria can be identified and specific treatment prescribed. The germ may be different with each infection, suggesting that the bacteria are invading from outside the body. If the same germ is found each time, it is possible that a stubborn focus of infection in the urinary tract is not being destroyed by the antibiotics.

Recurrent infection with the same germ can be seen in patients with infected cysts or kidney stones. All urinary tract infections in PKD patients should be treated aggressively and usually for longer periods than in persons with normal kidneys. Women patients with recurrent infections (who have reasonably normal kidney function) are advised to drink six to eight cups of fluid each day (preferably plain water), urinate every two hours during the day and within 30 minutes after intercourse. Evaluation by a nephrologist or urologist is also advisable.

Stones

Question: Can persons with PKD have kidney stones removed with the new shock-wave machines? Lyman, SC

Answer: PKD patients have a high incidence of kidney stones, and these can cause serious problems. A recent review of the use, in a number of medical centers, of extra corporeal shock-wave lithotripsy on PKD patients with stones suggests that it can be used with few complications.

Question: I am male, 38 years old, and was diagnosed with PKD in 1987. I have recurrent calcium oxalate stones for which I take hydrochlorothiazide twice daily, potassium citrate (12 tablets daily) and magnesium oxide. I pass three to five stones per week, all less than 3mm in diameter. I have normal amounts of oxalate in my urine and drink three to four quarts of water a day. Nothing seems to work. Will anything stop kidney stone formation?
Virginia Beach, VA

Answer: Stone formation can be stopped in most patients, including those with PKD, with simple measures such as drinking enough fluid and, when the chemical composition of the urine is abnormal, with dietary changes or medications such as those you are taking. You should realize that passage of stones does not always indicate that a particular treatment is not working. X-rays are needed to confirm that the stones that are passed are new and not stones formed before starting the treatment. The patients who fail the conventional types of treatment and continue to form stones may benefit from evaluation in centers specializing in renal stone disease.

Brain Aneurysms and Cysts

Question: My mother and her brother had PKD and both had ruptured brain artery aneurysms in their 50s. I am 42. Should I have an X-ray test for brain aneurysm?
Kansas City, MO

Answer: Current estimates indicate that *in the absence of any symptoms* the risk of a PKD patient having an aneurysm is between 5 percent and 10 percent. Aneurysms tend to run in families. Current studies suggest that there are no compelling reasons to screen *all* persons with PKD for aneurysm; however, if there is a family history of aneurysm, screening by angio magnetic resonance imaging (MRI) is indicated. Patients with PKD who note a *change in symptoms* involving the head region (blurred vision, dizziness, severe headache) should consult their physician. PKD Conference

Question: Can you please tell us symptoms of aneurysms of the brain and the abdomen. Boise, ID

Answer: Aneurysms (ballooning) of brain blood vessels will occasionally cause recurrent, severe headaches. Patients have also reported eye disturbances, nausea, vomiting, and stiff neck. Fortunately, aneurysm of the brain vessels is relatively uncommon. The aneurysms tend to occur within families of patients who have polycystic kidney disease. We all have headaches from time to time, so long-standing "nagging" headaches should not be a worry to patients with polycystic kidney disease. On the other hand, a PKD patient with a new type of headache that is unrelenting should seek medical attention. Aneurysms in the abdominal blood vessels usually occur in the aorta, the major blood vessel running through the body just in front of the spinal column. Patients will occasionally notice an "extra heartbeat" in the upper abdomen when an aneurysm is present. These types of aneurysms can also cause pain in the abdomen of a nonspecific nature. It is relatively easy to check for abdominal aneurysm with a sonogram test to exclude this as a cause for abdominal pain.

Question: I am a PKD patient on dialysis. Two weeks before my kidneys failed I had a stroke. The CT scan showed an intracerebral (brain) hemorrhage, but no aneurysm. I know about PKD and cerebral aneurysms, but I wonder if there is a connection between PKD and intracerebral vessel weakness? Seattle, WA

Answer: Individuals with high blood pressure, whether they have PKD or not, have a higher incidence of intracerebral hemorrhage than those who do not have elevated blood pressure. Since more than one-half of polycystic kidney patients have elevated blood pressure, there may be an increased incidence of stroke due to intracerebral hemorrhage that is not related to aneurysm formation. There is no information to indicate that the blood vessels of polycystic kidney patients are inherently weaker than normal. Thus, intracerebral hemorrhage in a PKD patient with normal blood pressure should raise the question of an occult cerebral aneurysm.

Question: I am 38 years old and recently had surgery to clip two aneurysms. Will I develop more and when should I be checked? Ann Arbor, MI

Answer: Currently, there is no information about when aneurysms develop in ADPKD, nor is there any information on if and when a person with an aneurysm should be rechecked. However, in people who have small aneurysms but do not have polycystic kidneys, physicians recommend follow-up studies at four- or five-year intervals.

Question: Once an aneurysm has been found, how successful is surgical intervention? Lawrence, KS

Answer: Not all intracranial aneurysms require surgery. While aneurysms causing symptoms should be treated immediately, the recommendation for surgery in the case of incidental, asymptomatic aneurysms will depend on the estimated risk of rupture if left untreated and the risk of surgery. These risks are determined by the number, size and location of the aneurysms, the age of the patient, and the expertise of the neurosurgeon. In good hands, the average incidental intracranial aneurysm can be repaired with a less than 5 percent risk of dying or having major complications.

Question: We have heard of patients with PKD who have ruptured a cerebral aneurysm. My husband has PKD and is 65 years old and on dialysis. His sister died of a ruptured aneurysm at age 32. We have three children ages 24-33 and the oldest has PKD. What if anything should we do? Dallas, TX

Answer: It does not appear necessary to look for aneurysms in every person with PKD since it seems that aneurysms are not very common in PKD. There has been a suggestion that aneurysms may occur in some PKD families and not in others. Because of this, some doctors might suggest that only PKD patients in such families, or PKD patients who would cause a high risk to others if an aneurysm ruptured and they became unconscious (like an airplane pilot) should be studied for aneurysms. Ruptured aneurysms don't seem to happen very often in PKD patients on dialysis. The tests available to look for aneurysms include arteriography, computed tomography, and the new technique of magnetic resonance angiography. This last test appears to be the easiest and the best.

Question: My husband, who has PKD, had a mitral valve replaced. Is he more susceptible to having a cerebral aneurysm since he has mitral valve prolapse and liver cysts? We have been advised by a physician that he is at increased risk even though he has no family history of aneurysm. What is the current recommendation regarding screening for aneurysm? Bartlett, IL

Answer: There is no evidence that PKD patients with mitral valve prolapse or hepatic cysts have a particularly increased risk of having an intracranial aneurysm. Some preliminary data suggest that patients with very severe polycystic liver disease may have an increased risk; this will require confirmation. The best noninvasive test to screen for intracranial aneurysms is magnetic resonance angiography. This test, however, is expensive and not widely available. A provisional recommendation, which is subject to difference of opinion, is to screen patients with a family history of intracranial aneurysms, patients with high-risk occupations such as pilots, patients planning to undergo major elective surgeries, and patients with severe or unusual headaches.

33

Question: My 38-year-old sister has been diagnosed as having two fluid-filled arachnoid cysts in the lining of the brain. A CT scan and MRI were used to confirm this diagnosis. The doctors don't know if these cysts are associated with PKD. Do you have any information about this? Ashland, MA

Answer: Arachnoid cysts have indeed been detected by CT scan in several patients with polycystic kidney disease. Very little is known about how these cysts in the brain may affect patients. In the experience of a few nephrologists, these cysts have been asymptomatic and no treatment was recommended. There is very little experience in the management of these cysts. Should a patient develop symptoms that neurologists and neurosurgeons agree may be caused by an arachnoid cyst, direct intervention may be indicated.

34

Pregnancy

Question: I'm 18 years old—diagnosed with PKD at birth. My creatinine level is 3.3. How might I go about having children without a complicated pregnancy?
PKRF Annual Conference

Answer: Assuming you are of normal adult height and weight, the creatinine level suggests that kidney function is between one-fourth and one-third of normal. If high blood pressure is present, both of the factors of a low kidney filtration rate and high blood pressure make pregnancy complicated and sometimes extremely difficult. Not only may there be complications that endanger health, but there may be complications that endanger the baby's health. Prior to pregnancy, it is very important to seek the advice and counsel of a "high risk" obstetrician; that is, someone who takes care of pregnant women who have complicated health problems. One should ask specific questions about the risks to the mother and to the baby. In autosomal dominant PKD, the child will have one out of two chances of having the disease; if the disease is autosomal recessive, the disease will not be passed on unless the father should have one recessive gene. At the moment there is no way to know about this in advance.

Question: I am a 28-year-old female with PKD. My creatinine is normal, as is my blood pressure. I have no obvious symptoms of PKD. I would like to become pregnant, but my husband and I are concerned about the stress pregnancy puts on a woman's kidneys. Would you recommend that I see a nephrologist before becoming pregnant?
La Mesa, CA

Answer: There is no evidence to indicate that pregnancy accelerates the progression of PKD in individuals who are asymptomatic and have normal renal function. A comprehensive assessment by a nephrologist (history, physical examination, and laboratory studies) is clearly indicated to determine the status of kidney function before pregnancy. Women who are normal, except for the diagnosis of PKD, have a good prospect for a successful pregnancy and the delivery of a full-term infant. Individuals with mild abnormalities in blood pressure and kidney function face increased risk of complications during pregnancy, and for those with moderate or severe problems, pregnancy may be contraindicated.

The decision of individuals with PKD to become pregnant is highly personal, and there are no "rules" in this respect. Once pregnancy is verified, it is important to visit a physician/obstetrician on a regular basis to monitor blood pressure and urine. Urinary tract infections should be treated promptly.

It seems that women with PKD are more likely to develop high blood pressure during pregnancy than women in general. It also appears that pregnancy increases the number and size of liver cysts. There is not agreement in all studies about the effect of pregnancy on kidney function. The most recent study suggests that three or more pregnancies may be associated with a decrease in kidney function over time.

Question: What is known about the potential effects of diet and toxic chemicals ingested during pregnancy on the formation of polycystic kidneys? North Hollywood, CA

Answer: Some information has come from the production of cystic disease in animals. Pregnant animals ingesting large doses of glucocorticoids (drugs such as prednisone) have offspring that have cysts in the kidneys. It has been thought that this might be due to the low blood potassium levels that occur when corticoids are taken, but we now know from studies of kidney tissue grown in a culture dish that application of glucocorticoids also causes cysts to develop. In addition, large doses of thyroid hormone will do the same thing. It should be understood, however, that this takes very large quantities of the drug; many women taking glucocorticoids have given birth to babies with normal kidneys.

There are a number of other chemicals that have been used to produce kidney cysts in experimental animals. Once again, large doses are required, and we have no information to suggest that any type of cystic kidney disease results from environmental toxins. It must be remembered that most cystic diseases (especially autosomal dominant and autosomal recessive) are inherited. It may be, however, that some drugs and toxins can accelerate the growth of cysts. Caffeine is one chemical that is recommended be eliminated from the diets of patients with cystic disease. It probably stands to reason that drugs be taken only when medically necessary and that one try to eliminate any large quantity of environmental toxin from the surroundings.

37

Kidney Failure

Question: I have PKD and am 46 years old. My parents are in their 60s and have no signs of kidney failure. What can I expect? Boulder, CO

Answer: It used to be felt that people in the same family had the same course of PKD. This does not seem to be completely true. We do know that some PKD families have a different gene than most other PKD families. This gene is called PKD-2 and causes kidney failure later in life. Except for this, the disease can progress differently within families. In recent information, it seems about half of all PKD patients are alive and without kidney failure by about 60 years of age. PKD patients with normal blood pressure seem to do better than PKD patients with high blood pressure.

Question: Does where you live have any effect on PKD? What causes the kidneys to slowly lose their normal functions? Dagsboro, DE

Answer: Several informal surveys have failed to show any tendency for polycystic kidney disease to be worse in one section of the United States when compared to another. As far as we can tell, the polycystic kidneys begin to lose normal function when the cysts become so numerous and large that they crowd out the normal kidney tissue. There is probably more to it than this, but most current evidence favors the view that the cysts simply distort the architecture of the kidneys and thereby cause them to function abnormally.

Question: One question that I have not gotten any answer for is how long it generally takes before the kidneys fail and dialysis is needed? Monrovia, CA

Answer: The progression of polycystic kidney disease to renal failure is highly variable. A recent study showed that only about 50 percent of patients with PKD will ever develop kidney failure that requires dialysis or transplantation. That is the good news! The bad news is that doctors cannot tell in the early stages of the disease who will and who will not develop kidney failure. Most of the patients who ultimately require dialysis or transplantation need this therapy by the age of 50 or 60. There are a number of exceptions, however, who have required dialysis at the age of 20, 30, or 40. In other words, there is not a simple, direct answer to your question. Nephrologists are relying now on the CT scan to give an estimate of the amount of normal tissue that is left in the kidneys at any point in time. It may turn out that this will be the best way of predicting the long-term outcome of kidney function.

Question: One nephrologist told me to drink at least 12 glasses of water daily. I tried the prescription but, having to void every hour was inconvenient. I am now drinking about six glasses of water. What is the appropriate fluid consumption for patients with polycystic kidney disease?
Pompano Beach, FL

Answer: There is no exact response to your question on how much fluid one should drink. We usually encourage patients to drink as much water as they feel they need to drink to satisfy thirst. Some patients with polycystic kidney disease are unable to fully concentrate the urine and therefore require more water than others. Twelve glasses of water per day (three quarts) sounds a bit excessive. We would suggest that for those patients who do not feel compelled to drink water, 1-1/2 to 2 quarts of total fluid per day is probably sufficient in most cases. Of course, patients who receive dialysis treatments must follow a rigorous fluid and diet prescription ordered by their physician.

Question: I read with interest your article in *PKD Progress* in which you suggested that patients with PKD should refrain from using caffine. As a dietitian who occasionally counsels patients with PKD, this sparked my interest. Would you be able to provide me with references?
Van Nuys, CA

Answer: Experiments that are currently being conducted in research laboratories indicate that drugs such as caffeine and theophylline could accelerate cyst formation in patients with PKD. Both of these drugs are known to increase within kidney cells the level of a compound called cyclic AMP that causes increased rates of cyst enlargement. There are no clinical studies, however, that prove or disprove that caffeine or theophylline affect the rate that kidney cysts expand. Nonetheless, it seems appropriate to alert patients to the possibility that these substances could potentially have harmful effects on polycystic kidneys.

Question: Would you comment on the desirability of a patient with PKD having penicillin prophylaxis at the time of dental care? North Whitefield, ME

Answer: Patients with mitral valve prolapse (approximately 30 percent of ADPKD patients) should probably receive dental prophylaxis with penicillin or another antibiotic. In the absence of this condition, however, prophylaxis is not recommended at the time of dental care unless the patient is receiving dialysis treatment.

Diet

Question: In view of the finding from the MDRD study that a low protein diet does not slow the progression of PKD, are these diets still recommended for individuals who have not reached the dialysis stage of the disease? Ames, IA

Answer: While the low protein diet study has failed to show clear benefit, dietary management can still be recommended to reduce symptoms in patients approaching end-stage renal disease, or in managing potassium and phosphate retention. For the purpose of slowing the progression of renal disease, certain individuals do seem to have a beneficial change in their rate of decline, although the overall study is negative. The best course of action is to work with your individual nephrologist and dietitian to find out what might be reasonable for you while still maintaining good nutritional status.

42

Question: I'm 46 years old and have had low back pain that I thought was from old football injuries, but I have just been diagnosed with PKD. My kidneys are enlarged and my liver has cysts. Occasionally after a workout, my urine is dark. What do you think? Should I follow a special diet? Address unknown

Answer: Chronic back pain is common in many people, and about 60 percent of all ADPKD patients have that complaint. You should inform your doctor of your symptoms of dark urine after exercise so your urine can be checked for blood. A *high* protein diet or extra protein supplements are definitely *not* recommended.

Question: Do we know what causes kidney cysts to enlarge, and are there any dietary or lifestyle modifications that can be made to prevent this from occurring?
Falmouth, ME

Answer: We know that for cysts to enlarge they need to make more cells and secrete more fluid into the inside of the cyst. Although we know some of the factors that can cause this in a "test tube," we do not know what causes this in people. Because a drug like caffeine can cause cysts to grow in a "test tube," it may be advisable to avoid large amounts of foods and beverages high in caffeine.

Question: My friend with PKD has been told to reduce the amount of protein in her diet, but she also has hypoglycemia (low blood sugar), which is treated by increasing dietary protein. Which condition should take priority in respect to dietary protein? Anderson, SC

Answer: Protein restriction has been used in an attempt to prolong the course of patients with established chronic kidney disease, including PKD. While the low protein diet study has failed to show clear benefit, dietary management can still be recommended to reduce symptoms in patients approaching end-stage renal disease.

Hypoglycemia is very rarely due to organic causes, but a skilled renal dietitian could give the best advice about the exact proportion of protein and carbohydrate, which must be in any individual's diet so that such coexisting conditions can be accommodated.

Drugs

Question: Have there been studies on the side effects of long-term drug therapy for hypertension—20, 30, 40 years? PKRF Annual Conference

Answer: Blood pressure lowering drugs have been used now for more than 30 years, and while there are some theoretical adverse effects on patients of different antihypertensive medications, these theoretical risks are markedly outweighed by the advantage of better blood pressure control on cardiovascular health.

Question: It is my understanding that there is a drug in the experimental stages for use on patients with polycystic kidney disease. I also understand that its use on some animals has proven to eliminate the cysts in those affected with the disease, but that the amount of the drug needed to do this is far too great for any human to tolerate. What can you tell us about this type of research? Bunkie, LA

Answer: Research is being conducted to find drugs that will slow the progression of renal cysts in patients with polycystic kidney disease. This kind of research is done in a multistep process. The first step in the sequence is to use test tube models of cysts to screen potential drugs for the effect of slowing the growth of the cysts. Several candidate drugs have been found in the test tube experiments to have an effect of slowing the rate at which cysts grow. Some of these are being tested in experimental animals, but there are no results to report. These types of studies often take several years to clearly validate whether a drug may or may not be worthwhile. When one or more candidate drugs are found, they will be tested in individuals with polycystic kidney disease in a strict research protocol, and they will not be offered to the general public for treatment until efficacy and safety have been clearly established. In summary, there are currently agents in the "pipeline" that are promising, but the use of these drugs in human beings is several years in the future.

Question: I am 68 years old; five years ago I began using nifedopine for a heart problem. Since that time my creatinine has risen from 2.0 mg/dl to 6.0. Is there any information on the use of nefedopine in PKD? Marquette, MI

Answer: There is no information on nefedopine in ADPKD. Although some medications can affect kidney function, nefedopine has not been reported to be a problem in patients with ADPKD.

Question: Are there any known effects of hormones on PKD cysts? Address unknown

Answer: There are no known effects of hormones on kidney cyst formation in patients. However, there is a growing body of data that female steroid hormones, both those which rise naturally during pregnancy and perhaps those which are taken in the form of birth control pills or postmenopausal estrogen, may affect cyst growth in the liver. Pregnancy appears to be one of the major determinants of liver cyst number and liver cyst size, making women particularly likely to develop large numbers of liver cysts. The role of birth control pills and postmenopausal estrogens are less clear. Birth control pills contain very low doses of estrogen compared to the amount of estrogen exposure that one receives in pregnancy.

Question: A patient with polycystic kidney disease is taking sinemet and synthroid and feels that cysts seem to be growing faster since the medications were started. Could these medications have any effect on cyst growth? Lanesville, IN

Answer: There is no specific information regarding these two drugs causing enhanced growth in patients with PKD. It is theoretically possible that either of them could do this in a laboratory environment, but no specific studies are available.

Question: Do beta blockers such as labetolol have any history of enlarging polycystic kidneys? Harrisburg, PA

Answer: There is no evidence that beta blockers or other anti-hypertensive drugs cause enlargement of polycystic kidneys.

Question: I have arthritis in my thumb joints and my doctor advises me to take only acetaminophen. Will aspirin hurt my polycystic kidneys? Mt. Laurel, NJ

Answer: Acetaminophen or aspirin in usual doses for short-term indications has no major impact on kidney function. Long-term use of combination analgesics can produce kidney damage, which would be in addition to that already present in polycystic kidney disease. The best advice is to limit the amount of analgesic that is used. If the need is prolonged, these drugs should be prescribed under the direct supervision of a physician who can carefully monitor the patient for adverse effects and who can maintain excellent blood pressure control.

Question: I frequently use propoxyphene for lower flank pain. Will this damage my polycystic kidneys?
Agana, Guam

Answer: Propoxyphene is frequently used as an analgesic for pain from PKD. This drug has not been studied alone for its adverse effects on the kidney. Combination analgesics containing aspirin, phenacetin, acetaminophen and caffeine have been most associated with long-term kidney damage. The use of any single ingredient for a prescribed period of time probably will do no serious damage to the kidney, but if pain and discomfort are prolonged, chronic pain management should be scrutinized by a nephrologist.

Question: Is there any known effect of lead exposure on a person with PKD, such as earlier onset or more severe illness? Helena, MT

Answer: Lead exposure, particularly in childhood, can lead to kidney disease in the absence of polycystic disease. If a patient has underlying abnormalities, obviously any lead-induced kidney damage would be additive. There are ways to test whether a patient's total body lead burden is increased. If this is proven to be the case it might make sense to use chelating drugs to lower the lead content of the body. The possibility of lead exposure should be evaluated by a competent specialist in nephrology or occupational medicine.

Pain

Question: I've heard that with laparoscopy, a technique that enables surgeons to operate on internal organs through tiny incisions, kidneys can be removed. How does that affect the viability of the tissue for research? Is there any room for the use of this technique in the management of PKD?
Salt Lake City, UT

Answer: Laparoscopy has been used on an experimental basis in the management of polycystic kidney disease. Under a grant from the Polycystic Kidney Research Foundation, investigators at Oregon Health Sciences University are reducing the volume of cyst fluid through the laparoscope in patients with refractory pain and discomfort from their polycystic kidneys. Should this technique prove feasible and safe, wider indications for active intervention in established cystic disease could be possible. It would be difficult to completely remove large polycystic kidneys through a laparoscope. For this, standard surgical techniques are probably necessary.

Question: Is there an analgesic (pain killer) of choice for the PKD patient? Millville, NJ

Answer: This is a difficult problem for PKD patients that has been made even more problematic by a report in the *New England Journal of Medicine* that suggests that acetaminophen may injure the kidneys if taken for long periods of time. It appears, therefore, that no analgesics can be used with impunity. Codeine and other narcotics can lead to dependency or addiction. Non-steroidals (aspirin, ibuprofen, naproxyn and several more) can reduce the flow of blood through the kidneys and aggravate high blood pressure. Acetaminophen can probably be used in small doses for short periods of time without injuring the kidneys, but patients with chronic, severe pain may have to consult a specialized pain clinic in order to consider alternative types of treatment.

Question: I am 36 years old and I have very painful polycystic kidneys. Doctors say the kidney function is normal. I have a stone in one kidney. I feel constantly tired and ill. A surgeon removed some of the larger cysts, but that did not help. Now he is considering cutting the sympathetic nerves to the kidneys. Can you tell me if this is normal for PKD patients and if there is anything else that can be done? West Sussex, England

Answer: Your situation is shared by others with PKD, but fortunately pain of this severity is limited to fewer than 10 percent. It is very difficult for doctors to pinpoint the exact cause of severe chronic pain in most cases, but occasionally kidney stones, kidney infections, kidney bleeding, blockage of the drainage tubes or kidney tumor may be found and corrected. We do not know the cause of pain in those individuals without obvious cause. We suspect that there may be inflammation in the kidneys caused by the cysts, but this is only a theory at the present time. Some patients get relief from an operation that removes hundreds of cysts from the kidneys, but this treatment has not been widely applied in the United States. Others have been helped by clinics that specialize in the management of chronic pain through biofeedback, transcutaneous stimulators and local injections of pain-killing drugs. If these measures fail it may be necessary to resort to analgesics, but many of these may potentially damage polycystic kidneys (acetaminophen, aspirin, and ibuprofen). This is an area of PKD management that continues to frustrate patients and physicians.

Cyst Aspiration

Question: A 64-year-old patient with polycystic kidney disease on dialysis has enlarged kidneys and liver that are so large as to be very uncomfortable. A recommendation has been made that one of the kidneys be removed, but the patient still passes one liter of urine per day. Is cyst aspiration an alternative? Springfield, MO

Answer: Cyst aspiration can be performed in any modern radiology department using ultrasound guidance. It is reasonable to try to aspirate large cysts in the kidney and liver to ascertain whether or not this will provide pain relief. If relief is obtained, the procedure can be repeated at intervals. If pain recurs frequently, a surgical procedure can be done to reduce cyst volume, although in a dialysis patient it may make more sense to simply remove the kidney. The presence of adequate urine output would seem to dictate a try at the aspiration technique prior to any consideration for kidney removal.

Question: Does surgery or puncture of cysts preserve kidney function in patients with ADPKD? And what are the indications for this procedure? Lincoln Park, NJ

Answer: Thirty years ago it was thought that surgery or drainage of cysts was associated with a more rapid decline in kidney function than would otherwise have occurred. Recent experience at Oregon Health Sciences University and the Mayo Clinic have suggested that kidney function is *not* adversely affected by these procedures, and in selected cases might actually improve it, particularly if the procedures are done relatively early in the course of the disease.

Often, blood pressure control improves, at least for a period of time. The major benefit of the procedure is to relieve pain and discomfort if they are severe and disabling to the patient. The operation, if skillfully performed, gives a high level of relief of these symptoms. It is customary to perform aspiration of cyst fluid under ultrasound to see if the patient obtains any relief prior to resorting to surgery. It should be emphasized that patients who do best with surgical reduction of cysts are those in whom the symptoms are so bad that their lifestyle is markedly affected. This type of surgery should be done by surgeons familiar with the techniques involved.

Sports

Question: A young patient has polycystic kidney disease and has recently traumatized his kidney while playing softball, which required eight days in the hospital. The patient still wants to play baseball and basketball. Should he wear any special protection, or simply avoid these sports? Richmond, VA

Answer: This is a difficult issue. It makes sense for patients with polycystic kidney disease to avoid contact sports such as football and ice hockey, in which direct trauma to the back and abdomen is likely to be sustained. Basketball also can lead to injuries like this, although this is less likely. It would not appear that baseball or softball would make a patient especially prone to kidney injuries. Protection is imperfect in avoiding these types of injuries, and may not be practical in baseball or basketball. Thus, the decision as to whether to participate in any sport is an individual one. In general, it is best to try to have the patient live as normal a life as possible. If this sport is necessary for psychological well-being, it might be reasonable to try it after a discussion of the pros and cons with your nephrologist.

Dialysis

Question: I have been on dialysis four years and am doing well except for unrelenting kidney pain. I am interested in having a transplant, but I want a better quality of life if I go to the trouble. Would it be best to have my diseased kidneys taken out before the transplant? Mahopar, NY

Answer: This is one of the most common issues facing PKD patients who are awaiting transplants. Opinions vary among transplant physicians and surgeons regarding the need to remove all polycystic kidneys before transplantation. Some surgeons insist that all kidneys be removed before the transplant, whereas other equally successful surgeons remove the kidneys only if there is evidence of infection, persistent bleeding, tumors, stones, excessive size or debilitating pain. Until recently, one reason to leave the old non-functional kidneys in place was their capacity to make a hormone that keeps the red blood count relatively high.

53

Erythropoietin has been approved by the FDA for use in anemic dialysis patients. This hormone will improve blood counts in anemic dialysis patients and improve the way they feel. Thus, PKD patients can have their kidneys removed without fear of developing debilitating anemia. On the other hand, if the old PKD kidneys have continued to make significant amounts of urine (more that 500 cc per day) dialysis patients will lose this amount of extra water they can drink if the kidneys are removed. Thorough discussion among members of the transplant team and the patient is indicated in each case before pretransplant nephrectomy is done.

Question: I am a 70-year-old dialysis patient with cysts in the kidneys and liver. Can I have these cysts surgically removed without recurrence? New York, NY

Answer: Unless your kidneys are giving you a great deal of pain or other problems, such as infection, it would be unwise to have them operated on simply to remove some of the cysts. Your kidneys are probably making a hormone called erythropoietin that will help keep the red blood cell count elevated. Patients with PKD generally have higher blood counts on dialysis than patients with other renal diseases. Occasionally, it is necessary to remove the kidneys if they become extremely large, painful or have excessive bleeding or infection problems. If you have none of these problems, it would be of no advantage to remove either the individual cysts or the kidneys.

Question: Is there anything a polycystic kidney patient being treated with chronic ambulatory peritoneal dialysis can take to increase the blood pressure? Fresno, CA

Answer: Patients with all types of kidney diseases who are treated with dialysis, peritoneal or hemodialysis for chronic kidney failure occasionally experience periods of low blood pressure. Polycystic kidney patients do not seem to be singled out in this respect. Most commonly, low blood pressure is caused by the loss of body fluids due to aggressive dialysis or because of intercurrent problems such as vomiting or diarrhea. In a few individuals, the blood pressure may be persistently decreased despite adequate attention to body fluid status and the elimination of medications that might lower the blood pressure. Nephrologists will usually test for heart failure, nerve damage (neuropathy) or the interposition of other diseases such as amyloidosis or Addison's disease in the search for the cause of hypotension. Unfortunately, there are a few individuals in whom no cause can be found and the nephrologist must resort to a trial of different medications that may be of benefit.

Question: What advice can you give on the care of arteriovenous grafts used for hemodialysis? New York, NY

Answer: Grafts are tricky things. Some become clotted early and repeatedly. Others remain open for years. They become clotted for a number of reasons—too much pressure on them (particularly if you lie on that arm at night), decreased blood pressure, abnormal clotting mechanisms, and strictures that develop in the veins at the end of the grafts, to name a few. Many of these things are beyond control. Individuals should not allow prolonged pressure on the graft or too tight clothing on that arm, for example. Blood presssure should not be taken in that arm, unless the person taking it knows a lot about grafts and has no other option but to take it in that arm. Very importantly, it helps to adhere to the fluid management plan between dialyses to avoid gaining a great deal of fluid weight. The fluid ingested between dialyses gradually seeps into the tissues. During dialysis the fluid must come out of the blood vessels before any can move from the tissues. The blood volume then becomes very low, and may lead to clotting. Sometimes blood thinning agents are prescribed for those who have repeated clotting, especially when no strictures are found in the graft.

Question: Has any research been done concerning the stimulation of sweating both as a form of dialysis and as a means of shedding excess water gained during peritoneal dialysis? Milwaukee, WI

Answer: Yes. Several years ago an imaginative manufacturer of sauna equipment proposed that sauna-bathing might be an effective way to control uremia and water retention in individuals whose kidneys had failed. A subsequent study showed that sauna-bathing (sweating) did not work. While metabolic poisons and water are lost in sweat, they are lost in amounts that are too small to affect the progression of uremia or over-hydration. Sweating is not an effective or efficient substitute for dialysis.

Question: A patient with polycystic kidney disease is on hemodialysis. She has restless legs at night, which are painful. It is questioned whether or not this is something that is common in polycystic kidney disease. Dallas, OR

Answer: Restless legs are generally a sign of neuropathy (nerve irritation) in patients with chronic renal failure on dialysis. They are not specific to polycystic kidney disease. Since they occur in patients on dialysis from other causes, the patient's nephrologist should be consulted as to whether the dialysis prescription is appropriate to maximally provide relief of neuropathy symptoms.

Question: I have polycystic kidney disease and I'm on dialysis, and I wonder if enlarged kidneys cause severe diarrhea? Lake Wylie, SC

Answer: Although there is no published information on this subject, physicians who care for large numbers of PKD patients occasionally find some with chronic diarrhea. In these few patients diarrhea appears to be related to the function of the nerves that control movement in the intestinal tract and not due to kidney size.

Question: I am a PKD dialysis patient. I have incessant nausea, which my doctor feels is caused by the liver and kidney cysts. Is there anything to relieve the nausea? Rochester, NY

Answer: Patients on dialysis may have nausea for a variety of reasons, such as insufficient dialysis, too much acid production by the lining of the stomach, or neuropathy caused by the renal failure. A markedly enlarged polycystic kidney or liver can press on the stomach. As a result, patients may feel full with small meals, have frequent heartburn, and vomit easily. These organs can compress the inferior vena cava (the vein returning the blood to the heart), which can cause low blood pressure during dialysis, and may be associated with nausea. Without having a better idea about the cause of your nausea, we cannot give you more specific recommendations. Sometimes physicians cannot find or solve the cause of the nausea and antinauseant medications are prescribed.

57

Transplantation

Question: When a patient receives a kidney transplant, what happens to the polycystic kidneys? Do they interfere with the new kidney? Utica, MI

Answer: At present, differences of opinion exist on whether the polycystic kidneys should be taken out before kidney transplantation. In the last 10 years, the most common practice has been to leave the kidneys in, unless they are massively enlarged, have been infected, or cause pain, recurrent bleeding or severe hypertension. There are several reasons for this practice. The surgery to remove the polycystic kidneys is very extensive and has a significant risk of death of up to 5 percent in some studies. In addition, there is no guarantee that the renal transplant will be successful, and patients on dialysis who have had their kidneys taken out have in the past often required multiple transfusions for severe anemia. But some nephrologists now find the argument for taking the polycystic kidneys out prior to transplantation more appealing because of improved success rate of renal transplantation, the elimination of anemia associated with renal failure with erythropoietin treatment, and some reports of severe hemorrhages and infections in polycystic kidneys not removed before transplantation. Nevertheless, in answer to your specific questions, most polycystic kidneys do not grow or become smaller after transplantation and do not interfere with the new kidney. Until more information becomes available, it seems reasonable to continue the current practice of leaving in painless, non-infected polycystic kidneys of moderate size prior to transplantation, but the pros and cons of this decision should be carefully weighed with each individual patient.

Question: Isn't a kidney transplant the only "cure" for polycystic kidney disease at the present time? Lenexa, KS

Answer: There is no cure for PKD. When the kidneys no longer function adequately, renal dialysis and kidney transplantation are treatments for this disease that have been used successfully for more than 20 years. The kidneys fail in about 50 percent of individuals with PKD. Dialysis of blood or dialysis by the peritoneal route is a lifesaving treatment when the kidneys fail and can be adapted for long-term use. The success rate of dialysis in PKD patients is among the best for all renal diseases that cause kidney failure. Many PKD patients elect to have a kidney transplant. Most of the donor kidneys come from non-related persons (cadavers) since one-half of the relatives of an affected patient also have PKD. PKD patients who receive kidney transplants do as well as those with other diseases. Current success rates indicate that more than 80 percent of kidney transplants will be functioning one year after the operation.

59

Question: Will polycystic kidney disease attack a newly transplanted kidney, and what is the survival rate of transplants in patients with polycystic kidney disease? Port St. Joe, FL

Answer: There is no evidence that polycystic kidney disease occurs in a transplanted kidney. This is expected since ADPKD is inherited and a transplanted kidney would not be likely to contain the genetic abnormality. Survival rates following kidney transplantation in patients with polycystic kidney disease are similar to all other patients undergoing transplantation. In fact, 80 percent to 85 percent of kidney recipients can expect a one year survival of the kidney transplant from a cadaver donor.

Living related donors can be used in polycystic kidney disease patients if the donor is shown to be free of the disease. Results from living related donors approach 90 percent to 95 percent one year graft survival.

Question: Can an unaffected sibling of a patient with ADPKD approaching the need for dialysis or transplantation serve as a donor? Jefferson City, MO

Answer: If a prospective donor who is greater than 21 years of age has a completely normal CT scan or ultrasound, he/she is very unlikely to carry the gene for ADPKD. If the prospective donor showed any cysts when a teenager, he/she likely carries the gene. A positive ultrasound or CT scan now as an adult would confirm the diagnosis. A negative ultrasound as a teenager does not exclude the diagnosis. While there is no certainty at age 21 that cysts, if present, will be large enough to be detected, most physicians are comfortable that a negative ultrasound and CT scan at this age means that the gene was not transmitted and donor evaluation could proceed. In the course of that evaluation, DNA testing could add a final degree of certainty that the donor does not carry the ADPKD gene, but at least two members of the family must be affected by ADPKD for the gene test to be informative for the prospective donor.

Question: Should a cadaver kidney transplant be performed in a patient with ADPKD prior to the need for dialysis? Marion Center, PA

Answer: Transplantation with kidneys from recently deceased, unrelated persons is frequently performed on PKD patients and is as successful or more successful than cadaveric transplants in general. Many transplant centers do not like to perform transplants or put patients on the cadaveric transplant waiting list until their renal disease is advanced enough to require dialysis. This policy has multiple reasons, not the least of which is the shortage of cadaver donor organs for people who are already waiting on dialysis. Also, it is often a good idea to have a trial of dialysis since many patients feel much improved and thus go into transplantation psychologically better prepared to face the 15 percent to 20 percent rejection rate of cadaver organs.

Question: A PKD gene has been located on chromosome 16. Can you tell me why that gene would not affect a transplanted kidney? Middletown, NY

Answer: We do not know how the abnormal gene on chromosome 16 causes cysts to form in patients with polycystic kidney disease, but if polycystic kidney disease is caused by an abnormal substance in the blood, one might expect that cysts would form in a kidney transplanted from a non-related person. The experience of many transplant surgeons and nephrologists indicates that cystic disease does not recur in kidneys transplanted into polycystic patients from individuals who do not have polycystic kidney disease. This "experiment in nature" shows that polycystic kidney disease does not recur in a non-related transplanted kidney and that polycystic kidney disease is probably not due to an abnormal factor circulating in the blood.

Question: A patient with advanced polycystic kidney disease requires a kidney transplant. Her 39-year-old sister has only two small cysts in the liver and none in the kidney (shown by contrast-enhanced CT). Would she be an

acceptable donor of a kidney for her sister?
Des Moines, IA

Answer: This is a difficult question. It is most common to find kidney cysts develop before liver cysts. Liver cysts do occur, although infrequently, in the general population. If this individual's liver cysts were numerous and large, one would be hesitant to recommend that she donate a kidney. If this family had other affected members and could be tested for PKD-1 by gene linkage analysis, that would be the first step to try. If gene testing is not a possibility, one could look for other markers of PKD in the potential donor's sister, such as inability of the sister to concentrate her urine when she does not have access to water, looking for other extra-renal signs of PKD such as mitral valve prolapse and the presence of hypertension. If the sister who is a potential donor has high blood pressure, inability to concentrate her urine, or mitral valve prolapse, that would increase the likelihood that she has the gene and makes her a less likely donor.

Question: My dad has PKD and I also have the disease. I am the only child of four who has been diagnosed as having the disease. Can I have a kidney from one of my sisters or brother if needed? Address unknown

Answer: Each of your sisters and brother has a 50/50 chance of having inherited PKD as you did. Patients older than 20 years of age will exhibit PKD when examined by computed tomography scanning (CT scanning), when the test is done with contrast enhancement. This is the most sensitive diagnostic test we know of with the exception of the genetic linkage test. In a family with PKD, the genetic linkage test can determine whether asymptomatic individuals have the gene, irrespective of whether or not the X-ray tests show positive. Unfortunately, this gene test is only available in a few genetic counseling centers in the United States.

General Information

Question: Those of us with PKD and decreased kidney function hope for a cure. My question is: Who can expect to be saved from kidney failure by a PKD cure?
Los Angeles, CA

Answer: All of us in PKRF are both working for and hoping for a cure for this disease. We can't predict when the cure will come or what it will be. However, the earlier people are in the course of the disease and the healthier they are, the more likely it is that some new treatment will work for them. Therefore, everyone should try to keep themselves and their kidneys in good shape with a healthy diet, regular exercise, by not smoking, and keeping their blood pressure under control.

Question: My father had PKD and he had strokes caused by his blood getting too thick. This was eventually treated by removing excess blood, after which he did fine. I have PKD and this worries me. Do you have an explanation?
Holly Springs, MS

Answer: The expression "the blood getting too thick" has been used to describe different medical conditions. In the case of your father, he likely had a condition called nephrogenous polycythemia. This is due to an excessive production by the kidney of a hormone named erythropoietin. Polycystic kidneys tend to produce this hormone in excessive amounts. Because of this, PKD patients have less problems with anemia than patients with other types of kidney disease when the kidneys fail. Very rarely the excessive production of erythropoietin, when the kidneys still have good function, is severe enough to cause polycythemia. Some medications, like water pills, can aggravate the polycythemia and should be avoided. As the renal function deteriorates, the production of erythropoietin decreases and the polycythemia disappears. The treatment of nephrogenous polycythemia is periodic removal of the excessive blood. Recently, physicians have found that a class of antihypertensive medications, the converting enzyme inhibitors, are helpful in reducing the secretion of erythropoietin and controlling the nephrogenous polycythemia, at least under some conditions. Although your father probably had nephrogenous polycythemia, this is a very rare condition and is not likely to affect you. You should be more concerned about preventing and, if necessary, treating other conditions that sometimes are also referred to as having "thick blood," that is, hypertension and high cholesterol.

Question: How do alcoholic beverages affect persons with PKD and liver disease? Laurel, MD

Answer: Although alcohol does not appear to have adverse effects on kidney function, it would seem advisable for PKD patients to restrict use to one or two ounces per day. Alcohol can increase uric acid production and in this way increase the risk of kidney stones. For someone with liver disease, alcoholic beverages of all types and in any amount are potentially harmful.

Question: I have several simple cysts in my kidneys. What causes these cysts? Is there any treatment? Groton, SD

Answer: Simple kidney cysts develop in about 50 percent of individuals over the age of 50 years. They are **not** inherited like autosomal dominant PKD or autosomal recessive PKD, but develop from microscopic kidney tubules (called nephrons) in much the same way that hereditary cysts form. These tubule segments expand progressively and fill with fluid, and sometimes reach the size of a hen's eggs or oranges. They can be confused with renal tumors and cancers, but they are otherwise usually harmless. In some uncommon cases, it may be necessary to operate on the kidneys to rule out cancers or remove an infected cyst, but in most cases no treatment is needed.

Question: If one kidney is removed from an individual with PKD, will the cysts in the other kidney grow faster? Cochrantown, PA

Answer: Many patients with PKD have had one of their kidneys removed because of infection, stone, tumor or accidental injury. Experience has not indicated that the remaining polycystic kidney grows any faster than it might have were the other kidney left in place. As indicated previously in *PKR Progress,* it is difficult to judge just how fast the polycystic disease will progress in an individual. Only about one-half of those with PKD will develop kidney failure in their lifetime; the remainder may have few complications of the disease. Thus, when a kidney is removed from an individual, one does not know whether that person was destined to develop renal failure or not. Nephrologists are very reluctant to remove polycystic kidneys from individuals with good to moderate levels of renal function. On the other hand, for those already en-rolled in a chronic dialysis program or who have received a successful renal transplant, nephrologists are more likely to recommend removal of polycystic kidneys that are causing discomfort or other medical complications.

Question: Do you know what causes cysts to grow so

rapidly in some people and what can be done to slow their growth? Massillon, OH, and Salem, OR

Answer: Some patients with hereditary PKD develop very large kidneys early in life that may progress to renal insufficiency over a quicker time frame than others in the same family. The nagging question is why this condition can be so variable among individuals even within the same family. We suspect that there are both hereditary and environmental factors involved in the formation and enlargement of kidney cysts. Researchers have not turned up any dietary substances that might be implicated in causing cysts to grow at a faster or slower rate. In research laboratories, however, some progress has been made. It is possible to make test tube models of kidney cysts grow faster by treating them with certain growth factors such as insulin, epidermal growth factor (a substance that causes premature tooth eruption and eyelid opening in newborn mice), and hormones such as antidiuretic hormone, prostaglandin, and drugs that inhibit an enzyme called phosphodiesterase (theophylline, caffeine). By contrast certain drugs such as ouabain, amiloride, ethacrynic acid and bumetanide can slow the growth of the cysts in the test tube. This means that it is possible that cyst growth in polycystic kidneys may be governed by similar types of substances. We hasten to point out, however, that none of these drugs and hormones have yet been shown to have any effect in animals with polycystic kidney disease or in human beings with the disorder. Research is currently going on to determine if hormones and drugs can alter the rate at which cysts expand in animals with hereditary types of polycystic kidneys.

67

Question: I have PKD with relatively few symptoms. When I visit my nephrologist once a year, what should I be asking and writing down to keep track of my condition over the years? Address unknown

Answer: Although there are many aspects of ADPKD that you could track, it is probably most helpful to document your blood pressure and your renal function with a serum creatinine. In fact, it is probably desirable that you monitor your blood pressure more often than once a year and share the information with your doctor. Although it is not necessary to have regular ultrasound examinations, any-time one is performed for a clinical reason it would be good to note kidney size and know whether there are cysts in other organs.

Question: I understand PKD patients can dehydrate quickly as said patients do not "concentrate" their urine. Would you please explain? Artesia, CA

Answer: Several studies have shown that in the intermedi-ate stages of the disease, PKD patients cannot maximally concentrate their urine. This is usually shown by determin-ing the concentration of salts in the urine after withholding water for 18-24 hours. In PKD patients, the cysts cause defects that prevent the kidney from maximally conserving water during even mild water restriction. This will some-times show up as nocturia, the need to get up and empty the urinary bladder two or three times during the night. Intercurrent illnesses are even more problematic since PKD patients may become dehydrated when they have high fevers or diarrhea or vomiting, because the kidneys cannot optimally conserve water.

Question: I was recently diagnosed with PKD; my twin sister also has PKD, but hers is farther along than mine. I wonder if individuals with PKD are prone to certain body shapes. All of a sudden my sister is barrel-shaped with a large body and skinny arms. I have seen others with kidney disease look this way. Are we more prone to this body shape as the disease progresses? Springvale, ME

Answer: There is no known body habitus associated with PKD. It is possible that patients with rapidly enlarging kidney and liver cysts might appear to be barrel-shaped because of the size of the cysts. Also, fluid retention in the abdomen can cause a shape that looks like this. A physical examination by a knowledgeable physician might provide the explanation for your sister's appearance.

Question: What is the average life expectancy for an individual with the adult form of PKD? Falls Church, VA

Answer: The life expectancy of individuals with the adult form of PKD is much better than thought years ago. In general, this is due partially to milder forms of the disease being diagnosed more frequently, better preventive medicine and medical care, and to the success of dialysis and renal transplantation. For these reasons, the estimated mean life expectancy of PKD patients in a recent study approaches that of the general population, while it was 15 years shorter in older studies.

Question: Are there dangers to a PKD patient flying in an unpressurized airplane? Encino, CA

Answer: The dangers to a PKD patient from flying in an unpressurized airplane as a passenger are not different from those to an individual without PKD. Because of the increased risk for intracranial aneurysms, it has been recommended that PKD patients fly an airplane only with or as a copilot.

Question: I have PKD. Everyone in my family has adult onset, but all kids check out okay. I know my children will have a 50/50 chance of having it, but it's more likely to be adult onset. Can you tell me what the chances are of them having childhood onset? Also, if they get it either in childhood or as adults, what percentage of cases are kept fairly well controlled with blood pressure medication, diet, etc., and what percentage end up with dialysis? How often does it progress to its worst before old age? What I am trying to determine is the quality of life and life expectancy that my children will have. I do not know if it is fair to have children knowing I carry this. Walkerton, IN

Answer: You are right, each child of an affected person has a 50/50 chance of getting the disease. Although most people with the disease don't have symptoms until adult life, some small percentage of children will have evidence of the disease in utero or shortly after birth. Many of these children do well. Children (one year of age or older) who have a parent with PKD often are studied with ultrasonography. Eighty percent to 90 percent of those children who have inherited the gene will have cysts before age 30. Children whose cysts are discovered in screening and who are otherwise well are likely to have a course just like people who are diagnosed as adults. That means that about 50 percent of them will be alive without kidney failure by age 50. The outcome is likely to get even better as we learn of the disease in utero or shortly after birth. Many of these children do well.

Question: I am 31 years old and have polycystic kidneys and liver. Although my CT scan shows almost no normal kidney tissue, my doctor says my blood tests of kidney function are normal. How can I find out what to expect for the future? Ellicott City, MD

Answer: You ask one of the most common questions posed to doctors who treat PKD patients. Unfortunately, there is no way to tell in a specific patient how long the kidneys will function adequately. Overall, only about 50 percent of PKD patients will ever require dialysis or transplantation, but that information can't be applied to a specific person. Some doctors rely on the CT scan done with dye contrast enhancement to judge prognosis (the future of function). Patients who have relatively large amounts of kidney tissue that show up with the dye seem to have a better chance of staying off of dialysis for several years than those whose kidneys have been nearly completely replaced by cysts.

Question: Why do some PKD patients develop distended abdomens and others don't? Does it have anything to do with the location of the kidneys (lower/higher)?
PKRF Annual Conference

Answer: The distention of the abdomen in some patients with polycystic kidney disease is caused by extremely large polycystic kidneys, polycystic liver, or both. The reason why some patients develop more severe enlargement of these organs than others is not known. Of interest is that polycystic liver disease tends to be more severe in women than in men, while polycystic kidney disease is slightly more severe in men than in women. Certain body configurations, obesity and, rarely, fluid accumulation can also contribute to abdominal distention in some patients with large polycystic kidneys or polycystic liver.

Question: What is the effect of exercise on polycystic kidneys? Should it be a routine? Should it be eliminated due to the stress? Flushing, MI

Answer: Moderate exercise is not harmful to polycystic

kidneys, unless the individual is experiencing urinary tract bleeding or infection. Under those circumstances bed rest or limited activity is usually prescribed. For individuals who have no symptoms, exercise is an essential part of a healthy lifestyle. Most individuals with PKD can engage in golf, tennis, swimming, walking or jogging. The key word here is *moderation.*

Polycystic kidneys are unable to normally concentrate the urine at certain stages in the evolution of the disease. Consequently, individuals should not subject themselves to prolonged periods of dehydration as may be experienced in long distance running, cycling or hiking.

Another reasonable rule of thumb is "if it doesn't hurt, it is probably okay." In other words, exercise programs that are moderately rigorous and do not cause discomfort in the kidneys are unlikely to cause problems. Once an individual encounters a symptom such as bleeding into the urinary tract or pain over a polycystic kidney, it is probably wise to eliminate that particular exercise from the routine.

The question of participation in contact sports has not been answered. Some renal specialists think that football, wrestling, boxing and other sports where direct injury to the kidneys might be incurred, should probably be avoided. On the other hand, there are other equally knowledgeable professionals who do not think that contact sports should be avoided in young individuals with no symptoms of their disease. Unfortunately, a carefully controlled study of this question has not been done, and physicians must rely on their experience and judgement in making recommendations in individual cases.

Question: We have a strong family history of PKD. My eldest sister has just been diagnosed as also having diabetes. Is this in any way a condition that is common in PKD patients? Bournemouth, Dorset, England

Answer: PKD patients do not appear to have an unusual incidence of diabetes mellitus. Diabetes mellitus can cause kidney problems that may aggravate the underlying PKD condition. It is a good idea for patients with both conditions to seek consultation with endocrinologists (diabetes specialists) and nephrologists to construct a treatment plan that can be monitored periodically by the team of physicians, and modified as newer therapies of these two disorders become available.

Polycystic Kidney Disease in Children ADPKD/ARPKD

Question: What kind of cystic diseases do children have?
Sacramento, CA

Answer: There are four major kinds of cystic disease that can be seen in infancy and childhood. The most common kind is called "multicystic dysplasia." It may occur in only one kidney or both and is frequently associated with an obstruction or absence of the ureter (the tube leading from the kidney to the bladder). It may be seen in children with some kinds of congenital malformation syndromes or may be an isolated entity. It is *rarely* inherited.

The second most common cystic disease in childhood is autosomal recessive polycystic kidney disease. In this disease, each parent carries one abnormal gene that, when matched together, lead to the production of many cysts. This occurs in both kidneys. The parent carrying the gene does not have the disease. *Each* child conceived by that couple has a 25 percent chance of inheriting the defective genes and, thus, having the disease, each has a 50 percent chance of inheriting one gene and being a carrier, and each has a 25 percent chance of inheriting neither gene and being normal.

Children with recessive PKD may be severely affected in that they are born with large kidneys, small lungs and, frequently, high blood pressure. Such infants often die because of lung problems. If the lungs are normal, however, the blood pressure can usually be successfully treated, and kidney function often remains good for many years. Some children require kidney transplants by late childhood or adolescence.

Recessive PKD also has an associated liver disease called congenital hepatic fibrosis. In some children this is mild and causes few problems; in others, the liver becomes very enlarged and causes increased pressure in the blood vessels surrounding the liver.

Thirdly, children may have autosomal dominant PKD. Now that screening procedures, such as ultrasound, are fairly sensitive, children in families known to have ADPKD may be found to have cysts, even though there are no associated symptoms. In a few children, high blood pressure and decreased kidney function can be seen early, rarely even in infancy.

In the very young child, the differentiation between 75 dominant and recessive PKD may be difficult. In those circumstances, a careful family history and ultrasound testing of the parents are very helpful. Sometimes a liver biopsy to look for the associated congenital hepatic fibrosis is necessary.

The fourth kind of cystic disease occasionally seen in childhood is uremic medullary cystic disease, sometimes called familial nephronphthisis. It is also inherited as a recessive disease, but is quite uncommon. Children with this disease usually have great hunger for both salt and water, may have nystagmus (the eyes flicker back and forth), and kidney failure usually occurs by mid to late childhood. Often these children are extremely anemic.

It has been thought in the past that any kind of

cystic disease, and particularly the inherited kinds, were all extremely severe and that children with these diseases would not live very long. We now know that is not true. Pediatric nephrologists believe that with careful attention to these children, treating complications as they occur, kidney function may remain good for many years.

Question: What are the qualifications of a pediatric nephrologist, and does the pediatric nephrologist differ from a regular pediatrician? Address unknown

Answer: The word "nephros" means kidney in Greek. Hence, the pediatric nephrologist cares for children with kidney diseases. This is in contrast to the pediatric urologist who is a surgeon who deals with operable conditions of the genitourinary tract, including congenital anatomical abnormalities and obstructions to urine flow.

A general pediatrician receives three years of training in pediatrics following medical school. In general, they have one to several months in which they care for children with kidney diseases, but they must rotate through all other subspecialties (such as neurology [nervous system diseases] and neonatology [newborn medicine]) as well as spend time caring for children with routine pediatric problems. The pediatric nephrologist spends those three years in the same way, but then has an additional two to three years in which he/she cares only for children with kidney diseases in order to learn extensively and intensively about the diagnosis and management of such diseases. General pediatrics has a "board" exam following the first three years. Passing that exam qualifies the doctor to be a "board-certified pediatrician." Pediatric nephrology also has a certifying examination that may be taken after the two- to three-year fellowship. The doctor then becomes a "board-certified pediatric nephrologist."

Question: Should my child with PKD go to a pediatric nephrologist? Address unknown

Answer: PKD in children is an uncommon disease. Pediatric nephrologists have trained in major pediatric centers that have large referral areas, so the pediatric nephrologist sees several children with PKD during training. On the other hand, the pediatrician-in-training might see only one or no such patients. Obviously, then, the pediatric nephrologist knows far better how to care for such children. If there is no pediatric nephrologist in your area, it is perfectly appropriate to ask your pediatrician to send your child for a consultation with a pediatric nephrologist in a university center. The consultant will then help the pediatrician plan an appropriate management strategy and educate the pediatrician on the ways to observe your child.

Question: Why does polycystic disease affect a fetus so quickly and fatally while it takes an adult years? Waco, TX

Answer: The quick answer is, we don't know. Medical research has revealed recently, however, that in the rapidly fatal type of recessive PKD, nearly all of the kidney tubules are altered by cyst formation. By contrast, in the adult autosomal dominant form only a small percentage of the tubules are affected with cysts. It may be that each cyst must grow to a much larger extent to cause damage when they are few in number, thus delaying kidney malfunction in the adult.

Question: If a couple has lost two children with infantile polycystic kidney disease and has one healthy child, will there be any chance that the healthy child will develop problems later in life—or will the parents develop problems? PKRF Annual Conference

Answer: Each child born of parents who carry one recessive gene each for ARPKD will have a 25 percent chance of inheriting both genes and consequently inheriting the cystic disease, or a 50 percent chance of being a carrier of one defective gene. If the child is normal at birth, does not have enlarged kidneys, and develops no problems with the kidneys or liver during childhood, there is little likelihood of later development of the recessive type of polycystic kidney disease. Although most children with ARPKD have enlarged kidneys at birth, a few will not develop detectably large kidneys or liver until later in childhood. High blood pressure may also be seen.

If the disease is suspected or if ARPKD is known to occur in a family, the young patient can be examined by sonography to determine if the kidneys and liver are normal. There are no reports in the medical literature to indicate that either parent of an affected child will ever show the recessive type of PKD. In other words, a solitary recessive gene in a carrier parent will not express the abnormality.

Question: In 1960 our son was born with infantile polycystic kidney disease and died eight days after birth. At that time little was known about this disease and it was never mentioned that it was inherited. The years 1961 and 1962 brought us two healthy sons. I wonder if infantile polycystic kidney disease is the same as the disease that strikes the 40- to 60-year-old group; therefore, is it a possibility that my two sons could develop polycystic kidney disease? Ann Arbor, MI

Answer: Research indicates that children with ARPKD may live well beyond the neonatal and childhood periods. However, these patients nearly always have some obvious evidence of polycystic kidney or liver abnormalities, and individuals 20 to 30 years of age with ARPKD would be aware of abnormalities in their kidney or liver function.

Thus, it is unlikely that your two sons have the infantile or recessive form of PKD. If there is any question, however, this could be checked by a consulting nephrologist. There is no evidence that the gene that causes the adult autosomal dominant form of PKD is in any way related to the gene that causes the autosomal recessive type of PKD.

Question: My daughter was born with adult PKD and I carry it. (I am under no treatment at this time.) She just turned six months and it breaks my heart that this happened to her. She is the only one of 13 offspring in our family who this happened to at birth. Why? Dearborn, MI

Answer: The autosomal dominant (adult) type of PKD is present at birth in the kidneys of individuals who have inherited the gene, but the degree to which the cysts are expressed varies greatly from person to person. With the almost routine use of sonography (sound wave testing) during pregnancy, many more cases of PKD are being discovered in unborn children. If the cysts are discovered in the fetus or newborn baby as an incidental finding (that is, no symptoms directed the physician to look for the disease), the outlook is no different than for anyone with the autosomal dominant type of PKD. However, recent studies of children in the University of Colorado polycystic kidney research program have indicated that early in life some children with ADPKD may develop problems.

If a child with PKD develops signs or symptoms, treatment should be started immediately and followed with regular health checks. Affected children without signs or symptoms of PKD should have regular checks for high blood pressure and urinary tract infections.

Question: I have PKD as did my mother. My 8-year-old daughter was born with only one kidney, but the remaining one is of normal shape, size and function. We have not had any kidney tests done to look for PKD. Could the missing kidney be due to PKD and should we be taking any special precautions? Fort Washington, PA

Answer: Although dominantly inherited PKD (ADPKD) can often be detected in childhood, this condition is not ordinarily associated with congenital abnormalities such as solitary kidney, so finding only one kidney has no special significance. A solitary kidney is relatively common in the population at large and does not usually lead to serious problems of renal function. Occasionally, the kidney will excrete more protein in the urine than normal, and some researchers have suggested there may be a predilection to high blood pressure in individuals with only one kidney. ADPKD does not appear to progress at an unusual rate in individuals with only one kidney, but this information is based on studies of older individuals rather than children. It would seem reasonable to have a child with a solitary kidney examined by a pediatric nephrologist at periodic intervals to check the level of kidney function and to monitor blood pressure.

Question: A letter comes from a grandmother telling that both of her children bore children with cysts on the kidneys. One child had bilateral cystic disease with underdevelopment of the lungs and died on a respirator. The child in the other family had cysts only in one kidney and is doing well. Investigation of inheritance factors showed no specific inheritance. The first family is having a second child after being told of no inheritance pattern, and this fetus has cystic kidneys also. Understandably, the grand-parents do not understand how this has happened.

Answer: It is impossible to determine from the informa-tion given, but it is likely that the family with the child who succumbed from bilateral cystic kidney disease carries the genes for autosomal recessive polycystic kidney disease. In this disease, no inheritance pattern is generally found, because the carriers (those persons who have only one abnormal gene) are asymptomatic. Any child born to that union has a one-out-of-four chance of having the same disease. Thus, the second baby appears to have inherited the two abnormal genes, also. The baby from the second family might have the same disease, but far more likely has the disease called multicystic dysplasia. That disease is uncommonly inherited and very commonly affects only one kidney. Although future children should be checked for recurrence, it is unlikely to be seen in a family pattern. It is usually possible to tell from the ultrasound findings if the disease is one of multicystic dysplasia rather than polycystic kidney disease.

81

Question: Two of my grandchildren died shortly after birth due to infantile PKD. A third child is a bright, sociable 4-year-old, but she has cysts on her kidneys and liver, and has high blood pressure. I wonder if it would be possible, in this age of genetic engineering, to have one of the parent's genes altered to produce a pregnancy free of this disease? East Kingston, NH

Answer: Despite the advances in genetic engineering we

are not yet at the point where we can correct genetic defects. The first experimental trials of these techniques are under way and intense efforts are being made toward the goal of "gene therapy." Nevertheless, it will be some time before these techniques can be applied in inherited kidney disease—many technical hurdles need to be overcome. In the meantime, a genetic counselor will be able to help your son/daughter-in-law evaluate the risk of PKD in a future pregnancy.

Question: My six-month-old daughter died of a virus that affected her heart. An autopsy disclosed autosomal recessive PKD. We want to have other children. What is the life span of this disease? Is there any treatment, surgery, medication or diet that would have helped? Canadian, TX

Answer: The viral disease that your daughter had was a separate disease from the autosomal recessive polycystic kidney disease (ARPKD). ARPKD results in death in early infancy in about 60 percent of those who have it. Usually, these babies die from lung problems, but some of them may have kidney failure. The remaining children may do well for a number of years. Some develop kidney failure fairly early and require dialysis or transplantation, and most children need that kind of treatment by or during adolescence. One of the most common problems associated with ARPKD in the child who survives is high blood pressure. We believe that prompt and careful treatment of the blood pressure will help maintain kidney function longer. There is no specific treatment for ARPKD, so we are careful to treat all the symptoms of the disease as it progresses.

Since you are hoping to have more children, you may wish to talk to a geneticist about the disease. The likelihood that each future child might have the disease is one in four, or 25 percent. Prenatal ultrasound examinations can sometimes, but not always, detect the disease before birth, and ultrasounds done sequentially after birth will also help with early diagnosis.

Question: I just lost my first baby to "bilateral cystic renal dysplasia, polycystic kidneys." I was told by the doctor that this type is not a genetic disorder, just a mechanical fault. Are there really forms of PKD that aren't genetic or recessive? Warwickshire, England

Answer: Unlike the genetically transmitted polycystic kidney diseases (autosomal dominant and autosomal recessive), bilateral cystic renal dysplasia is a sporadic condition caused by abnormal development of the kidneys early in embryonic life. The cause of multicystic dysplasia is unknown and, in many instances, this kidney malformation may be associated with malformations in other parts of the body. The bilateral cystic dysplastic kidney is considered to be nonhereditary. However, there are documented cases of familial recurrence of bilateral cystic dysplasia, particularly if there is a family history of other urologic abnormalities present. In families without a history of renal disease, there appears to be a small (1 percent to 3 percent) risk of recurrence of this problem in subsequent children.

Question: We understand that there are some projects under way to study autosomal recessive polycystic kidney disease, the type that affects infants. Where do these stand and what has been learned so far? What can we do to help? Surrey, England

Answer: The road to understanding the abnormalities in ARPKD requires several approaches. If one could start at the beginning, one would look for the genetic abnormality that produces a disease, determine whether that genetic abnormality was a single one or one of several abnormal genes that produced several abnormal gene products, determine what the gene products were (the proteins made by the genes that caused the abnormality), then determine whether there were some environmental factors that contributed to formation of the cysts, and, finally, how to alter the one of many processes that were abnormal. Needless to say, such a stepwise approach would take a very long time. For that reason, it is important that several processes be studied simultaneously, a procedure that requires the expertise of several different investigators with several kinds of expertise.

For those who have children with ARPKD, researchers are starting a registry and relatively soon will need blood samples from your affected child/children as well as other family members. You may want to notify PKRF of your willingness to be involved in research so that we will be able to contact you as appropriate needs arise.

Question: A family wrote to ask if it were true that there were four types of autosomal recessive or infantile polycystic kidney disease and whether all affected children from one family would have the same type. This is a particularly worrisome question for those families who have a baby severely affected at birth who quickly succumbs.

Answer: In 1971, two geneticists named Blyth and Ockenden (*J. Med. Genet.* 8:257, 1971) described ARPKD in children seen in London. They separated the children into four groups. A "perinatal" group presented at birth with huge abdominal masses that were the enlarged kidneys. These babies died within the first six weeks of life.

Microscopic examination of their kidneys showed that 90 percent of the kidney tubules were cystic, whereas the fibrosis of the liver was minimal. A second "neonatal" group presented from one day to one month of age with large kidneys. The majority of these babies had also died within the first six weeks of life. Sixty percent of the tubules were cystic and the liver scarring was a little more obvious. A third "infantile" group presented from three months to six months of age and had both enlarged kidneys and an enlarged liver. The majority of these children developed kidney failure but not until several years of age. In addition, they had very increased pressures in the liver blood vessels (called portal hypertension). In these children, only about 25 percent of the kidney tubules were cystic. Finally, a group called "juvenile" presented in childhood under the age of 5. The predominant symptom in them was the enlarged liver, and portal hypertension was severe. Less than 10 percent of the kidney tubules were cystic.

85

Several other reports of children with ARPKD have suggested this separation, and several authors have suggested that the affected children from a single family will always present the same way. That is, if one child has the perinatal type, any future child in that family who has ARPKD will fit in that same group.

More recent information says that this is not always true. Two recent reports have made a point of noting that one child can present with the severe, perinatal form and another will not develop severe disease until several years of age. Among our patients are several families whose presentations fit different types. On the other hand, there are some families in which the group seems to "breed true." That is, the affected children fit in the same group.

Unfortunately, there is no way to predict in advance whether affected children will fall in the same or different groups. One needs to remember, however, that *each child* in an affected family has only a 25 percent chance of having the disease at all and a 75 percent chance of being normal.

Index